RECLAIM YOUR HEALTH

Learn how to overcome the most common chronic illnesses

CANCER

By Award Winning Author
DR HARRIS PHILLIP

Co-Author
KESZIA FABIEN BSC

Disclaimer

The publisher and authors are not responsible for any specific health needs that may require medical supervision. If you have underlying health problems or have any doubts about the advice contained in this book, please contact a qualified medical doctor or an appropriately trained healthcare professional. It is not intended as, and should not be relied upon as, medical advice despite having an author with 30+ years' experience in practice in the medical field.

The information contained within this book series, Reclaim Your Health: Learn how to overcome the 9 most common chronic health challenges in modern times, Cancer is not intended to be used in the place of your general practitioner's advice or your family doctor's advice. This book series is provided for general information only and to empower readers by providing them with relevant information on the disease in an easily digestible format, thus ensuring their visits with their healthcare professional are richer and more rewarding. It will go a long way in helping you understand the pathognomonic features of this commonly seen chronic conditions called cancer, and it will provide you with some usable tools which you can employ to protect yourself from the daily insults on our bodies.

CONTENTS

Foreword

By Professor Ali Nakash

While continuing with his 30+ years' experience in clinical practice, Harris has decided to sum up much of what he has gained from seeing and treating thousands, maybe millions, of patients with a myriad of medical problems over the years. In his summary, which has been compiled into a series of twelve chunk-sized books, the reader is provided with usable tools which are presented in a simple, readily digestible format to allow everyone to benefit. From the least medically inclined among us, to the nursing student, the pharmacy student, the nurse, the pharmacist, the midwifery student, the midwife, the medical student, and the trained doctor, whether junior or senior. In essence there are useful nuggets of easy-to-follow guidance for all.

In the first book in the series, he starts with a disease we all dread. Many including my wife call it that disease.... You certainly know the disease to which I refer, it is cancer.

Reading through the pages of the first book in this series, I was immediately impressed with the presentation. Such a complex condition was condensed into such simple and easy-to-follow guidance. Not only has he addressed cancer from its cellular level, but he has also extended the discussion to allow you, the reader, to appreciate plausible causative agents for this condition once it is initiated. He gives some insight into how the disease process flourishes, and towards the end of the book he addresses how we can make ourselves cancer-proof.

Making ourselves cancer-proof I find particularly interesting since it allows both medical and non-medical personnel to explore avenues through which they can empower both themselves and their patients as together we fight this dreaded disease.

In the other books of this series which are being completed, the approach is the same, whether it is addressing Alzheimer's disease, cardiovascular disease, diabetes, or the other chronic health challenges of our time. I am particularly impressed with the presentation, the relative simplicity, and the inherent usefulness of this series. This doubtlessly will not only empower, but also serve as a useful companion handbook on our journey to reclaiming our health.

Mr. Phillip is an award-winning author for his book, STOP! It's Not Too Late!: Adding Years to Your Life and Life to Your Years Using the BMS Model, a book which I call an encyclopaedic guide to healthy living. But in this book series I think he has outdone himself as he seeks to provide the tools that we all need to reclaim our health.

He has most definitely put his years of training and experience in capsule form through the various books in this series. Mr Phillip is a trained senior consultant obstetrician and gynaecologist and has displayed his abundance of knowledge through the ease with which he addresses the various chronic health challenges of our times.

This series, for me, represents an interesting and empowering piece of medical science which has been presented in a digestible format for even the non-medical personnel among us. I am therefore moved to make this bold prediction that once you start reading these books, you will find it difficult to stop because of the timeliness and appropriateness of their contents.

Introduction

Several years ago, I was employed as a teacher, which incidentally was my first professional job. While entering the classroom to deliver a biology lecture to a group of students at the Saint Andrews High School, who were preparing to write the General Certificate of Education examination (GCE or GCSE, as referred to in the UK), a young man who claimed he had no interest in Biology collected his books and was leaving the classroom to go to the library, as I entered to deliver the lecture. The lecture was designed to highlight the characteristics of living things and to help distinguish the living from the dead. I commenced the lecture with the statement, 'once one starts living, he/she starts dying'. Inherent in that statement is that both living and dying are processes. Even deeper is the realisation that what we refer to as life is simply a grant of two dates and a dash. Upon hearing this introduction, the young man made an about-turn and asked permission to attend my class. I did not convert him into a biologist, but he left the class much better informed. Today that young man is a politician. We are granted a date of birth and a date of death: between these two dates is the dash and that is the focus of this book, how can we extend the dash to delay our date of death. I prefer to look at the whole scenario as a rubber band that can be stretched between two points, the two points being the date of birth and the date of death. We can do nothing about our date of birth, that date is beyond our control, but if my analogy of a rubber band is fully understood, and since our date of birth cannot be seriously influenced by our action or inaction, for the rubber band concept to hold, it means that the dash can be extended and thus we can delay our date of death.

My paternal grandmother, for instance, lived to a ripe old age of 115 years. She lived a fully independent life, still being able to cook and care for herself in her 115th year. This is not widespread, I hear you say, and my response is why not? Do we have any skills, knowledge, or abilities in the current era to approach this lifespan and make it more of the expected norm as opposed to an occasional event?

It is with this burning desire that I have used my medical knowledge, gleaned in the field, as well as my extensive research, the skills of which I learned as a university student in organic and biochemistry at a top 10 USA university as I pursed a PhD degree in Biochemistry. This training not only provided me with the skills and tools which I needed to pursue the more inquisitive aspect of my person, but also has alerted me to the value of research. Thus, when faced with a challenging question, I revert to research to help me determine the answer.

In observing the lifestyle of my paternal grandmother, my 30+ years of medical practice, drawing on the knowledge gleaned through my research, and from my study in organic chemistry, leading to my Master's degree and my sojourn through the biochemistry classroom, I believe that we have an opportunity to delay the second date, the date of death, by stretching in rubber band style the duration of the dash. This is therefore the purpose of this book: providing tools, suggestions and basic information which will hopefully allow you to prolong your dash and live a more dynamic and healthier life, thus adding years to your life and life to your years.

I will aim to provide sections on each of the nine most common chronic ailments of our time, suggesting how best one can delay the effect of the insult on our bodies, hence allowing us to live a more complete, fun-filled life, a guide to which has been developed in one of my earlier books, about using the BMS approach, an award-winning book.

In this book series we will look at cancer, Alzheimer's, dementia and diseases of the brain, heart disease and strokes, diabetes, arthritis, obesity, chronic lung diseases, and chronic kidney diseases, hoping that this series serves as a useful handbook – guide, if you will – in understanding and defeating the most common chronic ailments affecting human beings on planet earth.

I know that you may be stunned: why has a trained obstetrician and gynaecologist got involved in the writing of books addressing various aspects of health, some of which may be remote from obstetrics (care of pregnant ladies during their pregnancy and childbirth and for the first 42 days after ending the pregnancy) and gynaecology (the branch of medicine which deals with the functions and diseases specific to women and girls, specifically those relating to the reproductive system)? To this my response is simple:

It is the only medical discipline which allows one to practise all the facets of medicine. It therefore means that any good obstetrician and gynaecologist, because of the demands on his scope of practice, needs to be above average in his knowledge of internal medicine, surgery, paediatrics, social and preventative medicine, care of the elderly, and neonatology. Hence my familiarity with these various disciplines and the related physiology has empowered me in the provision of this book series which I am hopeful will be an empowering tool to help many understand elements of their health, while simultaneously allowing them to know when things are wrong and therefore see the need to seek medical advice. Hopefully the message is that the earlier a disease process is found, the more options will be available for management and the more likely a full cure will be realised.

BOOK 1
CANCER

CHAPTER 1
Background

- What is cancer?

- Processes by which control can be lost

- Oncogenes

  - In gene variants/mutations:

  - Epigenetic changes:

  - Chromosome rearrangements:

  - Gene duplication:

- Tumour suppressor genes

- DNA repair genes

- Pause For Thought

- Take Home Nuggets

- Pages for making personal notes

Cancer Research UK claims that all cancers' combined incidence rates are projected to rise by 2% in the UK between 2023 and 2025. It further predicts that between 2038 and 2040 the rise in cancer cases will reach 625 cases per 100,000 people.

Even more frightening is the realisation that the change in cancer incidence rates since the early 1990s has increased by 12%. This is truly alarming despite our best efforts in the management of this condition. Personally, I have been involved initially in the preparation of chemotherapeutic drugs to fight cancer. During my master's degree in Organic Chemistry, I was involved in the modification of the imidazole ring of DTIC, by replacing the nitrogen in the imidazole ring with sulphur; the belief then was that this would reduce the toxicity of the DTIC molecule. The drug DTIC is used in the fight against some gynaecological cancers. At that time, I was focused on finding a cure for cancer. I graduated with the degree and left this project behind.

Much has happened since: we have more highly specialised centres, employed more focal training, and improved our imaging techniques as well as increasing inputs from various sectors, through the multidisciplinary team (MDT) approach, but the incidence continues to rise. It therefore seems that our current approaches are failing. Is there any hope? Or are we simply on a treadmill going nowhere – that seems an appropriate lament. One cannot help but feel that the traditional approach to cancer treatment, that is surgery, radiotherapy and chemotherapy, have failed and continue to fail us. Within this section we are not promising to cure cancer, but we hope to introduce you to useful nuggets of prevention and the need for early cancer detection and presentation. In fact, we can say with confidence that the earliest stage at which a cancer is detected, the better the chances of having it cured.

What is Cancer?

The adult human body is composed of about 100 trillion cells. These cells are under precise control by other body mechanisms which instruct them on, among other things, when to divide and when the division process (mitosis) should stop. Simply, in cancer this sort of control is lost. To get a clearer understanding of the process and keeping it sufficiently simple, cells of the body go through what is called a cell cycle. The cell cycle is composed of about five major phases: G0 or resting phase; G1which reflects cell growth; the S-phase in which DNA replication takes place; G2 in which the cell is prepared for mitosis or cell division; and finally, the M-phase in which cell division takes place. To ensure a normal cell cycle there is need for precise control at every step. A loss of this control leads to cells behaving erratically, that is they no longer obey the start and stop signals. This tends to lead to tumour formation. A tumour can be either benign or malignant. It is the malignant tumours that we call cancers. These cancers develop features that try to ensure their growth and continued development, for example, by a phenomenon called angiogenesis. These cancers send out signals which encourage the development of blood vessels in the area which results in nourishment of the cancer. These cells can then continue to develop. Cancer development starts at the cellular level; therefore, cancers can arise from any site around the body.

The body has developed an independent mechanism for fighting cancer which doubtlessly works, but with variable success.

Processes by which control can be lost

Proto-oncogenes normally help cells grow and divide to make new cells or to help cells stay alive. These proto-oncogenes will occasionally undergo changes called mutations, or there may be too many copies of this proto-oncogene. It may become activated when it is not supposed to be; at this point it is now called an oncogene, which can cause the growth of cancer. Interestingly, the main types of genes that play a role in cancer are oncogenes, tumour suppressor genes, and DNA repair genes. Cancer is often the result of changes in more than one of these types of genes within a cell.

1. **Oncogenes:** Oncogenes can be turned on (activated) in cells in different ways. Example:

    (a) **In gene variants/mutations:** Some people may have differences in the 'code' of their genes that can cause an oncogene to be turned on all the time. These types of gene changes can be inherited from a parent, or they can occur during a person's life, when a mistake is made when copying the gene during cell division.

    (b) **Epigenetic changes:** Cells normally have ways of turning genes on or off that does not involve changes in the genes themselves. Instead, different chemical groups can be attached to genetic material (DNA or RNA) that affects whether a gene is turned on or off. These types of changes may lead to an oncogene being turned on.

    (c) **Chromosome rearrangements:** Chromosomes are long strands of DNA in each cell that contains its genes. Sometimes when a cell is dividing, the sequence of the DNA in a chromosome is changed. This might lead to the relocation of a gene that functions as a type of 'on switch' next to a proto-oncogene: this would keep the gene turned on even when it shouldn't be. This new oncogene can result in the cell growing out of control.

(d) **Gene duplication:** Some cells may have extra copies of a gene, which might lead to them making too much of a certain protein.

2. **Tumour suppressor genes:** These are normal genes that slow down cell division or tell cells to die at the right time (a process best described as programmed cell death or apoptosis). When these genes don't work properly, cells can grow out of control, which can lead to cancer.

Inherited mutations in tumour suppressor genes have been found in some family cancer syndromes. They cause certain types of cancers to run in families. Most tumour suppressor gene mutations are acquired during a person's lifetime and not inherited.

3. **DNA repair genes:** These genes help fix mistakes in the DNA; or if they can't fix them, they trigger the cell to die, to reduce any problems caused by the mistakes. When there is an error in one of these repair genes, it can allow more mistakes to build up inside the cell. This may affect other genes which could lead to the cell growing out of control. As with other types of gene changes, changes in DNA repair genes can be either inherited from a parent, or acquired during a person's lifetime.

Examples of DNA repair genes include BRCA1 and BRCA2 genes. People who inherit a pathogenic variant (mutation) in one of these have a higher risk of some types of cancers, particularly breast and ovarian cancer among women.

Pause For Thought

- Think about what is happening with cancer.

- Are we mere stooges waiting to be attacked and taken down by cancer?

- Is our defence system against cancer functional?

- If we have a defence system against cancer, why do we get cancer?

Take Home Nuggets

- The development of cancer is complex and may be caused by different processes.

- Cancer may develop by the failure of certain control mechanism influencing cell growth.

- Cancer may result from gene changes called mutations.

- Cancer may result from environmental factors.

- Cancer may be the result of failures and faults in cells.

Notes

_____

_____

_____

_____

_____

_____

_____

_____

_____

_____

_____

_____

_____

_____

_____

_____

_____

_____

_____

_____

_____

_____

Notes

_____

_____

_____

_____

_____

_____

_____

_____

_____

_____

_____

_____

_____

_____

_____

_____

_____

_____

_____

_____

_____

Chapter 2
The Body's Defence System Against Cancers

- Pause For Thought
- Take Home Nuggets
- Pages for making personal notes

Our bodies have an army which it uses against cancers; however, many times that defence system fails because of numerous factors. We will explore the known defence systems of our bodies and factors which may cause them to fail in the fight to protect us against cancers. Understanding these factors will give us the ability to successfully beat cancer.

The development of cancer is a complex process which involves several stages. Interestingly, at each stage, there are natural mechanisms designed to protect against the development of cancer. Most cancers found in humans are induced by carcinogens which are present in our environment and even in our foods. Some substances present in our diet or synthesised in body cells can reduce the cancer-causing potential of these carcinogens. The mechanisms available vary between blocking, entrapping, or decomposing these carcinogens. There is a battery of tumour suppressor genes which, as their name indicates, suppress tumour proliferation. Carcinogens can also be removed from our cells. Damaged DNA in many cases is repaired. However, DNA is not always repaired, and this damaged DNA becomes fixed as mutations in dividing cells. It is these mutations in strategic locations which can induce tumour growth. Those strategically located genes relevant to this discussion are the activating proto-oncogenes and the inactivating tumour suppressor genes. The proliferating tumour cells must find a way to continue to proliferate and to spread beyond the initial tumour location, a phenomenon called metastasis.

Among the last barriers involved in the protection against cancer activity is the immune system. Here both innate and adaptive immunity is involved in anti-tumour activity. This anti-tumour activity involves the activity of a host of different types of white blood cells: natural killer T cells, macrophages, neutrophils, eosinophils; the cytokine pathway specific antibodies and specific T cytotoxic cells. Once activated, the neutrophils and macrophages can destroy tumour cells. They are also able to release free radicals such as reactive oxygen species which are capable of damaging RNA, DNA, and proteins when they build up in cells, eventually leading to cell death. Although many cytokines exhibit anti-tumour activity, their role in natural anti-tumour defence is not well established.

Pause for Thought

- Think of the development of cancer as a complex process with many causes.
- Genetic faults or errors is a factor.
- The body has a built-in defence system.

- Cancer overwhelms the body's defence system to be able to nourish and replicate itself.

- Through developing its own blood supply, it is able to proliferate and spread.

Take Home Nuggets

- Understanding the behaviour of cancer helps us in fighting the disease.

- Recognition of the body's own defence system helps in the fight against cancer.

- By cutting off the cancer's source of nourishment and reinforcing our body' defence systems, we may be more successful in defeating the disease process.

Notes

_____

_____

_____

_____

_____

_____

_____

_____

_____

_____

_____

_____

_____

_____

_____

_____

_____

_____

_____

_____

_____

Notes

_____

_____

_____

_____

_____

_____

_____

_____

_____

_____

_____

_____

_____

_____

_____

_____

_____

_____

_____

Chapter 3
Triggers

- Environmental factors
- Person innate factors
- Pause For Thought
- Take Home Nuggets
- Pages for making personal notes

As intimated in the introduction, the detection of a cancer at the earliest possible stage gives one the best chance for curing the disease; most purists would confirm that the best chance of fighting the disease is through the prevention of the condition.

In its simplest description cancer results from the abnormal growth of certain cells in the body. The obvious approach to its prevention is to determine what triggers this abnormal growth and to determine if there are any means by which the activation of this trigger can be prevented. It has long been known that cancer is caused by changes to DNA. Most cancer-causing DNA changes occur in genes. These genetic changes can cause genes involved in normal cell growth to cause abnormal cell growth and are referred to as oncogenes.

It must also be understood that the body has its own army to mount a fight against these aberrant cancer growths, but it seems that a successful fight is less likely under certain conditions. Among the conditions are environmental factors, and person innate factors.

Environmental Factors

Exposure to a variety of chemical agents in the environment is known to increase an individual's risk of developing cancer. Among them are benzene, asbestos, vinyl chloride, radon, and arsenic. Other risk factors include smoking and tobacco, both from an individual smoking, and from inhaling second-hand tobacco smoke. Obesity and weight are also associated with the development of certain types of cancers. It is believed that being overweight and obese is the second biggest cause of cancer. Let me quickly interject here that being overweight does not mean that you will develop cancer, but if you are overweight you are more likely to get cancer than if you are at a healthier weight. Your diet can also increase your risk of developing certain types of cancers. Eating a healthy, balanced diet can help to reduce that risk. Sunlight and ultraviolet radiation, and sunbeds increase the risk of skin cancers. Consumption of alcohol can also increase your risk of developing certain types of cancers. The less alcohol you drink, the lower the risk of developing cancer. Physical activity can indirectly reduce the risk for certain types of cancers. The more active you are, the more likely you are of having a healthy weight and thus reducing your risk of developing cancer.

Certain viruses – for example, human papillomavirus (HPV) – are associated with an increased risk of developing certain cancers as well as human immunodeficiency virus (HIV). In fact, it is believed that Kaposi sarcoma is caused by human herpesvirus 8 (HHV-8).

Though cancer can develop at any age, certain types of cancers are more common in the elderly. So, age seems to be a risk factor. The common- sense advice in all these environmental factors is to avoid or minimise exposure to these known risk factors.

Person Innate Factors

Cancer genes (faulty genes) can be inherited from our parents: for example, BRCA1 and BRCA2 increase the risk of developing certain cancers in individuals carrying these faulty genes. Changes in our hormone levels can also increase the risk of developing certain cancers.

A compromised immune system, from whatever cause, be it other illnesses or exposure to some therapeutic agents. It is known, for example, that individuals who carry the human immunodeficiency virus (HIV) are at increased risk of developing some specific types of cancers. The use of radiation to treat certain types of cancers is associated with the development of certain secondary cancers. Even widely used medications such as metformin have been linked to the development of certain cancers. In the case of metformin, the risk seems, as stated in May 2020 by the Food and Drug Administration, to be associated with higher than acceptable levels of the substance called N-Nitrosodimethylamine (NDMA) in some preparations of extended-release metformin. There is no evidence that the standard-release metformin tablets are associated with an increased risk of developing cancer.

So, what is NDMA? I hear you ask. It is a chemical which is formed as a by-product of some manufacturing processes. Very low levels can be found in chlorinated water, cured, or smoked meats, and malt beverages such as beer and whiskey. NDMA may also form when medications are stored. The International Agency for Research on Cancer classifies NDMA as a "probably carcinogenic agent (able to cause cancer) to humans" based on animal studies. These studies showed that high levels of NDMA (10,000 nanograms/kg/day) in dogs, rats and mice caused significant liver fibrosis and cirrhosis. These liver diseases then led to the development of liver cancer. There are no studies of the carcinogenic effect of NDMA directly on humans. The Environmental Protection Agency limits NDMA in water to 0.7 nanograms/litre. In one review of the extended-release metformin capsules manufactured by Amneal, it was found to contain up to 395 nanograms of NDMA.

It would therefore seem that the triggers for cancer are multifactorial, hence there may be no single approach to beating or arresting this condition. It would therefore seem a sensible approach to visit countries with the lowest incidence of cancer to determine how they are able to keep the incidence of cancer low.

Pause For Thought
- Early detection is the best chance for cure.
- Cancer is the result of abnormal growth of cells.

- Faulty genes caused by DNA changes contributes to cancer development.

- Environmental factors also contribute to cancer development.

- Person innate factors can also contribute to cancer development.

Take Home Nuggets

- Genetic factors play a role in the development of cancer.

- Environmental factors such as cigarette smoking also plays a role in the development of cancer.

- Obesity is associated with cancer development.

- Diet is also a contributing factor to cancer development.

- Sunlight and the use of sunbeds are associated with cancer development.

- Infections with certain viruses is associated with cancer development.

- Use of recreational drugs such as alcohol is associated with cancer development.

- Unfortunately, cancer is more common among older individuals which makes age a factor in the acquisition of some cancers.

- Luckily physical activity reduces the risk of cancer development.

Notes

_____

_____

_____

_____

_____

_____

_____

_____

_____

_____

_____

_____

_____

_____

_____

_____

_____

_____

_____

_____

Notes

Chapter 4
Prevention

- Countries with the lowest incidence of cancer

- What is the evidence on fucoidan?

- Pause For Thought

- Take Home Nuggets

- Pages for making personal notes

Countries with the lowest incidence of cancer

In our search for preventive measures to reduce the incidence of cancer, it seems sensible to visit countries with the lowest cancer incidence around the globe to determine how their lifestyles, foods and environment etc contribute to the lower incidence of cancer among its people.

A visit to Okinawa, Japan, takes us to a city with among the lowest incidences of cancer. A study of that population reveals the use of a slimy weed which has been credited as a primary cause for the record-low cancer rates in Okinawa, Japan. It was used with reported success to treat and prevent radiation sickness following the Chernobyl meltdown in Russia.

Although this weed is yet to be subjected to clinical trials, the Japanese medical community reports that they are inundated with reports of how this medicinal seaweed has helped thousands of patients in the fight against cancer.

There has been a raft of reports which suggest a plethora of new natural remedies that produce impressive results among Japanese patients.

Let us focus on the complex of polysaccharides (carbohydrates) found in brown seaweed, most commonly in an Asia-Pacific variety known as kombu or Laminaria japonica. The active agent is called fucoidan. The seaweed has been a dietary staple in Japan since the second century B.C. and in Okinawa, which has Japan's highest rates of kombu consumption. Okinawa's residents eat daily about 1 g of kombu which contains about 5 mg of fucoidan, and they enjoy some of the longest lifespans in Japan and the single lowest cancer rate in that country.

What is the evidence on fucoidan?

In the 1990s, scientists identified fucoidan as the primary immune-building substance in brown seaweed and started to study it.

In one case, researchers injected female lab rats with a known carcinogen that induces mammary tumours. They fed half of the rats a standard diet plus daily portions of brown seaweed containing fucoidan, and the other half were given a standard diet. The animals were monitored for 6 months. The fucoidan-fed rats developed fewer tumours than those which were fed the standard diet. 63% developed breast cancers vs 76% of those who were fed the standard diet. Secondly, the fucoidan-fed rats resisted the development of the tumours for longer periods of time. Those fed a standard diet developed tumours as early as 11 weeks following exposure to the carcinogen, whilst those exposed to the fucoidan remained tumour- free for 19 weeks.

It therefore seemed that fucoidan worked in two ways to reduce the incidence of tumours: (a) it delayed the manifestation of tumours; and (b) it reduced the number of rats which developed tumours.

In other studies, oral and intravenous doses of brown seaweed proved from 61.9 to 95% effective in preventing the development of cancer in rats implanted with sarcoma cells.

Fucoidan has been described as a very potent antitumor agent in cancer therapy after it inhibited the growth and spread of lung cancer in rats.

Further studies indicated that fucoidan combats cancer in multiple ways among which are: (1) it causes rapidly growing cancer cells (including stomach cancer, colon cancer and leukaemia) to self-destruct (a process called apoptosis); (2) it physically interferes with cancer cells' ability to adhere to tissue. This prevents the cancer from spreading to new areas; and (3) it enhances production of several immune mechanisms including macrophages (white blood cells that destroy tumour cells), gamma interferon (proteins that activate macrophages and natural killer cells), and interleukin compounds that help regulate the immune system.

Fucoidan has been shown to work synergistically with other anti-cancer drugs, and is found in a product called Modifilan. The product contains fucoidan, along with organic iodine and alginate – a natural absorbent of radioactive elements, heavy metals and free radicals.

Pause For Thought

- The incidence of cancer across all countries is not identical.

- Incidence of cancer in Okinawa, Japan is among the lowest in the world.

- The inhabitants to this area have a diet rich in brown seaweed.

- The active agent in brown seaweed is fucoidan which is an excellent immune building substance.

- Fucoidan is found to be particularly active against a variety of cancers.

Take Home Nuggets

- The lowest incidence of cancer in the world is in Okinawa, Japan.

- Natives have a high consumption of brown seaweed.

- Active agent in Brown seaweed is fucoidan.

- Fucoidan attacks cancer in multiple ways.

Notes

_____

_____

_____

_____

_____

_____

_____

_____

_____

_____

_____

_____

_____

_____

_____

_____

_____

_____

_____

_____

_____

_____

Notes

_____

_____

_____

_____

_____

_____

_____

_____

_____

_____

_____

_____

_____

_____

_____

_____

_____

_____

_____

_____

_____

Chapter 5
Early Detection

- The AMAS test
- Pause For Thought
- Take Home Nuggets
- Pages for making personal notes

Simple blood test for early detection – the AMAS test

As intimated in the earlier introductory pages of this section, the earlier a cancer can be detected, the better the prognosis for the individual who is so afflicted. In our fight against this modern and all too common condition, a focus on early detection of the condition would inevitably lead to higher cure rates.

I am therefore enthused with hope that there are brighter days coming with the emergence of this test called AMAS cancer test. AMAS stands for anti-malignin antibody in serum test. Malignin is a peptide found in people with cancer. If the antibody to this peptide is detected in the blood, it would mean that the peptide has been detected in the body and an immune response has been launched. Clinical studies have shown that the AMAS test is 95% accurate on the first reading, and up to 99% accurate after two readings.

This simple blood test can detect both precancerous and cancerous cells with up to 99% sensitivity. Though this test has been available for some time, its roll-out to the public has been slow, with its promotion heavily dependent on word of mouth. Though in recent times its promotion has been more aggressive, there is still a long way to go.

One does not need a doctor's permission to order the test. Anyone can order the AMAS test by calling 1-800-922-8378 and leaving your name and address to receive a free kit in the mail. The kit comes complete with material and the instructions you need to complete the test, as well as instructions for overnight shipping. Your doctor will need to order the blood sample and sign the analysis form. All tests are analysed in Boston. Anyone anywhere in the world can order the test. Shipping, though, may be a challenge, as samples sent from outside of the USA may need to be shipped in dry ice to ensure that a valid sample arrives in Boston. The analysis costs about USD 165, not including lab fees and shipping costs. Ordering the kit, though, is completely free.

The AMAS test detects the presence of cancerous cells but not their location. A positive reading therefore will require further testing to locate the cancer and to determine its stage. This, though, gives us a means of detecting a cancer earlier than the more widely used screening tools. More on this test can be found by visiting the website www.oncolabinc.com.

Pause For Thought

- Early detection of cancer gives the best prognosis.
- What is the value of the AMAS test?
- What is the AMAS Test?
- Why does it give hope?

Take Home Nuggets

- The earlier a cancer is detected the better the prognosis.

- AMAS Test is a simple blood test which has a sensitivity of 95% if positive in early detection of cancer.

- Sensitivity refers to the possibility of an individual having a condition if a test is positive.

- The AMAS test has a sensitivity of 99% after two positive results.

- AMAS is a blood test for the antibody to malignin, a peptide found in people with cancer.

Notes

Notes

_____

_____

_____

_____

_____

_____

_____

_____

_____

_____

_____

_____

_____

_____

_____

_____

_____

_____

_____

_____

_____

Chapter 6
Graviola, Nature's Gift

- Graviola(sour Sop)
- How does it work?
  - Cell death
  - Block metastasis
  - Scramble signals
  - ATP
- What the research says
  - Breast cancer
  - Liver cancer
  - Lung cancer
  - Pancreatic cancer
- Potential risks
  - Nerve damage
  - Low blood pressure
  - Low blood sugar
  - Faulty test
- Pause For Thought
- Take home nuggets
- Pages for making personal notes

Graviola (soursop)

I will address graviola which is described as a natural cancer killer. With the use of extracts from this plant, the future of cancer treatment and the chance of survival are encouraging.

Since the 1970s, the bark, leaves, roots, fruit, and fruit seeds of the Amazonian graviola tree have been studied in numerous laboratories with remarkable results.

It has been shown that extracts from the tree seek out, attack, and destroy cancer cells. Why is this finding not known? you ask. Big Pharma have been unable to duplicate the tree's natural properties with a patentable substance, hence they shut down this project and it was not made public. In 1976, the National Cancer Institute showed that the leaves and stem of this tree were effective in attacking and destroying malignant cells. Since then, there have been several promising cancer studies of graviola. The tree extract is yet to be tested on cancer patients. Graviola (botanical name: Annona muricata), also called soursop, is a fruit tree that grows in tropical rainforests. People have long used its fruit, roots, seeds and leaves to treat all kinds of ailments, including cancer.

Modern scientists have been studying the plant for 50 years. They see potential promise in graviola. They found it kills cancer cells in test tubes and in animal studies. What they don't yet know is if it works as a treatment for cancer in humans.

How does it work?

Graviola is believed to contain hundreds of chemicals called acetogenins (ACGs). These chemicals, in lab tests, kill many types of cancer cells. The fascination is not only that it kills cancer cells, but also that it causes no harm to healthy cells. They can even treat tumours that haven't responded to cancer medicines. This raises the possibility of treatment with minimal side effects.

The acetogenins extracted from graviola seem to work in different ways to kill, block or otherwise fight different types of cancers. The pathways include:

Cell death. Old or damaged cells die naturally, a process called apoptosis. Cancerous cells often evade apoptosis and survive. Graviola leaf extracts encourage cancer cells to undergo apoptosis and die.

Block metastasis. The process by which cancer cells spread is referred to as metastasis. Studies indicate that graviola extracts stopped cancer cells' growth in vitro and in lab animals and prevents them from metastasising.

Scramble signals. Cells receive messages from inside and outside the cell. Signalling pathways relay the messages. A mistake in one of these pathways can lead to cancer. Graviola blocks pathways that control the growth and life cycle of cancer cells.

ATP. Adenosine triphosphate is the energy currency used in body cells as a source of energy. Graviola is able to starve cancer cells from ATP, and these cells die as a result.

What the research says

Graviola use has been studied in many kinds of cancers. The findings have been promising. But graviola has not been tested in clinical trials on people to know the results.

Breast cancer. Graviola leaf extract has been shown to shrink breast tumours in mice. Graviola fruit extract has also been studied in relation to a protein called epidermal growth factor receptor (EGFR). This protein sits on the surface of cells and helps them grow and divide. Some breast cancer cells have too much EGFR. The cells grow faster and are harder to treat. Graviola blocked the growth of these cells.

Liver cancer. Graviola has been shown to cause cell death in liver cancer cells.

Lung cancer. Graviola leaf extract stopped the growth cycle of lung cancer cells.

Pancreatic cancer. A powder of graviola leaves and stems caused cell death in pancreatic cancer cells. Graviola also blocked signalling pathways that help pancreatic tumours spread.

There is much to be excited about the potential use for graviola in the treatment of cancer.

Potential risks

One can buy graviola pills and liquid online and in natural food stores. No one knows the best dose or how much is safe.

Possible harms from graviola may include:

Nerve damage. It may be associated with movement disorders, like Parkinson's disease, as tremors and movement problems were seen in some laboratory animals.

Low blood pressure. The use of graviola in patients prone to develop low blood pressure may be a concern as a drop in blood pressure may occur in animals and humans.

Low blood sugar. In patients on hypoglycaemic medications graviola can reduce blood sugar levels.

Faulty tests. One of the benefits of graviola may also lead to interference with imaging studies, since graviola stops our bodies from absorbing radioactive drugs.

We do not suggest the use of graviola in place of your regular anti-cancer therapy currently. We would recommend discussing this with your doctor.

Pause For Thought

- Graviola and its cancer fighting ability.
- All parts of this plant seem to have cancer fighting qualities.
- Being a naturally occurring plant, it can't be patented.
- Could this be the reason why it has not been rolled out as a treatment option in the fight against cancer?

Take Home Nuggets

- Every component of the Graviola plant has cancer fighting ability.

- Graviola grows in many tropical rainforests.

- Research has revealed the ability of components of this plant to attack cancer in many ways.

- It cannot be patented by drug companies as it is a naturally occurring plant.

- Graviola extracts are active against a variety of cancers.

Notes

_____

_____

_____

_____

_____

_____

_____

_____

_____

_____

_____

_____

_____

_____

_____

_____

_____

_____

_____

_____

_____

Notes

_____

_____

_____

_____

_____

_____

_____

_____

_____

_____

_____

_____

_____

_____

_____

_____

_____

_____

_____

_____

_____

Chapter 7
AHCC

- How does AHCC bring about a boost in the immune system?
- Pause For Thought
- Take Home Nuggets
- Pages for personal notes

This is a hybridised mushroom extract which reportedly destroys cancer cells whilst simultaneously providing powerful immune protection. Until recently this remarkable immune booster was only accessible if you lived in Japan. AHCC refers to activated hexose correlated compound which is available in the Western world and even on Amazon.

AHCC is an extract of a unique mixture of several kinds of medicinal mushrooms known for their immune-enhancing qualities. Dozens of rigorous scientific studies have now established AHCC to be one of the world's most powerful and safe immune stimulators in both in vitro animal studies and human beings. In some cases, it has been shown to prevent the recurrence of liver cancer, prostate cancer, ovarian cancer, multiple myeloma and breast cancer, with no dangerous side effects. In smaller doses AHCC can also boost the immune function of healthy people, helping to prevent infections and promote well-being.

As we age, our organs also age and become less efficient. Our immune system also becomes less efficient in conducting its role. One of the earliest responders in our immune system is the natural killer cells (NK cells in short). These NK cells attach themselves to the surface or outer membranes of cancer cells and inject a granule quite like a hand grenade into the interior of the offending cell. Once inside, the granule explodes and destroys the offending cell, be it bacteria or a cancer cell. Interestingly, it remains undamaged and can set out to find, attack and destroy another offending cell. Measurements of NK cells activity correlate well with one's chances of survival. It is therefore logical that any increase in NK cell activity will help treat, facilitate recovery from and/or prevent illnesses in human beings.

How does AHCC bring about a boost in the immune system?

Research published by respectable bodies such as the *International Journal of Immunology*, *Anti-Cancer Drugs* and *Society of Natural Immunity* has reported on the health benefits and safety of AHCC. It has been shown that AHCC consistently and effectively boosts immune function.

It is believed to bring about this immune-boosting function in several ways:

It stimulates cytokine (IL-2, IL-12, TNF and IFN) production, which stimulates immune function.

It increases NK cell activity by 300%.

It increases the formation of explosive granules in NK cells. This improves the NK cells' destructive ability.

It increases both the number and activity of lymphocytes, with a 200% increase in T-cells.

Interferon inhibits virus replication and stimulates NK activity. Furthermore, it increases the formation of tumour necrosis factor (TNF);

these are proteins which help to destroy cancer cells.

This multifaceted approach to improve one's overall immunity has profound health benefits.

3 g of AHCC per day significantly lowered the level of tumour markers found in patients with prostate cancer, ovarian cancer, breast cancer and multiple myeloma. This study also revealed complete remission in six of 11 patients, and there was a significant increase in NK cell activity in nine of 11 patients.

Pause For Thought

- What is AHCC?
- What is the source of AHCC?
- What are the uses of AHCC?
- AHCC provides a multifaceted approach to improve one's overall immunity with profound health benefits.

Take Home Nuggets

- AHCC destroys cancer cells.

- AHCC provides immune protection.

- AHCC is now more widely available, even on Amazon.

- It is a mixture of several types of medicinal mushrooms.

- Rigorous scientific studies have established AHCC as one of the world's most powerful and safe immune stimulants. It protects against liver cancer, prostate cancer, ovarian cancer, multiple myeloma and breast cancer with no dangerous side effects.

- At lower doses, it can boost the immune function of healthy people, preventing infections and promoting wellbeing.

- AHCC promotes the activity of natural cells and enhances the NK cell grenade like activity.

- AHCC increases the NK cells activity by 300%.

- AHCC increases the number and activity of the lymphocytes with a 200% increase in T-cells activity.

Notes

_____

_____

_____

_____

_____

_____

_____

_____

_____

_____

_____

_____

_____

_____

_____

_____

_____

_____

_____

_____

_____

_____

Notes

_____

_____

_____

_____

_____

_____

_____

_____

_____

_____

_____

_____

_____

_____

_____

_____

_____

_____

_____

_____

_____

Chapter 8
Lessons from the Puerperium

- Lactoferrin
- Other uses of lactoferrin
- Pause For Thought
- Take Home Nuggets
- Pages for personal notes

Lactoferrin is an iron-binding protein found in colostrum from breast milk. We have been taught about the value of colostrum, so let us reflect for a moment. We were made aware that colostrum provides us with the first defence against infection and disease, and it provides us with the first source of chemicals integral to the immune system. The role of the immune system is to conduct ongoing surveillance on the body cells, organ by organ, eliminating foreign substances, thus ensuring that whatever is in your body belongs there.

During pregnancy, the pregnant woman's immune system is downregulated, but once she gives birth, she produces colostrum, or the first milk, which is rich in lactoferrin and restores her immune system. Lactoferrin should therefore never be given to a pregnant woman. It may have some value, though, as an abortifacient.

What is significant about lactoferrin?

Lactoferrin has at least two specific immune-boosting functions:

It binds to iron in the blood, making the iron unavailable to cancer cells, bacteria, viruses and other pathogens which require iron to grow. Lactoferrin is able to bind iron and release it as needed under specific conditions. In doing this, it helps in preventing harmful oxidative reactions. This is a useful quality and renders lactoferrin a powerful antioxidant.

Lactoferrin activates specific strands of DNA that are useful for genes necessary for launching an immune response. This is the only protein able to perform this function, making it unique.

Lactoferrin also contains antibodies against a wide range of bacterial, fungal, viral and protozoal pathogens. In essence, lactoferrin corners cancer cells as well as pathogens, starves them and signals to the white blood cells their precise location where they can be found and destroyed.

Several studies of rats and patient case histories have documented the benefits of lactoferrin helping to combat many types of malignancies.

Other case histories reveal that lactoferrin has been able to reduce and sometimes eliminate the harmful side effects of the more conventional chemotherapy and radiotherapy anti-cancer treatment. Thus far it appears that lactoferrin is perfectly safe even in high doses.

Other uses of lactoferrin

- It contains an anti-inflammatory molecule which means it is helpful in alleviating pain as well as joint inflammation.
- It helps in lessening ocular disturbance.
- It is useful against Candida albicans.
- It has potent antiviral activity.
- 100 mg of lactoferrin nightly at bedtime can significantly improve your immune system and effectively fight against environmental toxins, and emotional and physical stressors.

Pause For Thought

- What is lactoferrin?
- Where is it found?
- Why is colostrum the first defence against infection and disease?
- What role does lactoferrin play in the immune system?
- The role of the immune system is to conduct ongoing surveillance on body cells.
- Lactoferrin restores the pregnant woman's immune system.
- Lactoferrin should not be given to a pregnant woman because of the possibility of inducing an abortion.
- Lactoferrin is a unique protein.

Take Home Nuggets

- Lactoferrin is an iron binding protein found in colostrum.

- It is involved in providing the first defence against infection and disease.

- Lactoferrin plays a role in in restoring the pregnant woman's immune system.

- Lactoferrin should never be given to a pregnant woman because of the possibility of inducing an abortion.

- Lactoferrin has two specific immune boosting functions (1) it binds to iron in the blood, making it unavailable to cancer cells, bacteria, viruses, and other pathogens which require iron to grow. It is a powerful antioxidant; (2) Lactoferrin activates specific strands of DNA that are useful for genes necessary for launching an immune response. It is unique in being the only protein able to perform this role.

- Lactoferrin corners cancer cells as well as pathogens, starves them and signals to the white blood cells their precise location where they can be found and destroyed.

- Lactoferrin is also able to reduce and eliminate the harmful side effects of the more conventional chemo and radiotherapeutic cancer treatment.

- Lactoferrin combats pain associated with inflammation, lessens ocular disturbances, is active against candida albicans and it has potent antiviral activity.

- 100mg of lactoferrin at bedtime significantly improves the immune system. Lactoferrin also fights against environmental toxins and emotional and physical stressors.

Notes

_____

_____

_____

_____

_____

_____

_____

_____

_____

_____

_____

_____

_____

_____

_____

_____

_____

_____

_____

Notes

_____

_____

_____

_____

_____

_____

_____

_____

_____

_____

_____

_____

_____

_____

_____

_____

_____

_____

_____

_____

_____

_____

Chapter 9
The Value of Caesium Chloride as an Anti-cancer Agent

- Caesium Chloride
- Side effects
- Pause For Thought
- Take Home Nuggets
- Pages for personal notes

In the 1930s, the German Dr Hans Nieper began using caesium chloride to treat his patients. Dr Keith Brewer expanded this approach by combining caesium chloride with dimethyl sulfoxide (DMSO). Caesium is nature's most alkaline metal, and when combined with DMSO it directly targets cancer cells, stopping the metastasis of the cancer, stopping the associated pains, and shrinking the tumour mass. Caesium chloride is particularly useful as an anti-cancer agent in that it disturbs physiology. Most cancer cells require large quantities of glucose to grow and multiply. To get more glucose the sodium/potassium pump is integral. The sodium/potassium pump must run up to twenty times faster to provide adequate amounts of glucose to the cancer cells. The sodium/potassium moves sodium out of cells and potassium into cells. Caesium behaves to the pump as potassium, and once the caesium enters the cancer cells it blocks the channel and potassium can no longer leave the cell. It blocks the supply of glucose, and the cancer cells die.

DMSO is a super solvent. It can penetrate all cells, but attaching the DMSO to caesium allows for more specific targeting of cancer cells.

In April 1981 in Maryland, Dr H E Sartori treated 50 patients with caesium. The patients had widespread metastatic diseases of various primary cancers such as breast, colon, prostate, pancreas, lung and liver. In this study half of the patients survived, including three patients who were comatose when the treatment was commenced. Thirteen of the patients died within the first two weeks of commencing treatment, but autopsy revealed the tumour mass had reduced in size.

In the 1980s experiments with caesium led to the conclusion by the American Cancer Society that the use of caesium chloride led to less tumour growth and fewer deaths.

Caesium chloride and DMSO can be used either topically or orally; unfortunately, there are a raft of side effects associated with caesium use, so my advice is to avoid trying to use it without the supervision of an experienced and trained practitioner.

Side effects

Caesium can lead to hypokalaemia, so it would be necessary to take supplemental potassium. It must also be noted that caesium stays in the body for months so it would be necessary to continue potassium supplements for several months.

The combination of caesium with DMSO can cause the death of many cancer cells at once. The body's ability to process and eliminate this load of dead cells may lead to flu-like symptoms akin to a detoxification reaction. In rare cases, if taken as capsules, caesium can lead to perforation of the stomach or small intestines, if the capsules become positioned against the walls of either of these organs.

Pause For Thought

- Caesium chloride interferes with the physiology in cancer cells.
- It blocks the Na/K pump by mimicking the potassium. This effectively cuts off the much-needed glucose supply of cancer cells.
- DMSO is a super solvent, so when combined with caesium it allows for more specific targeting and destruction of cancer cells.
- Caesium is effective even against advanced stage cancers originating in the breast, colon, prostate, pancreas, lung and liver.
- Caesium is associated with numerous side effects and should not be used unless under the supervision of an experienced practitioner.

Take Home Nuggets

- Caesium is nature's most alkaline metal.
- Caesium attacks cancer cells by disturbing their physiology.

- It blocks the sodium/ potassium pump and interferes with the cancer cell glucose supply.

- When combined with DMSO, it is better able to target cancer cells. It is successful even in treating advanced disease.

- Its use is associated with several side effects and therefore, it should only be used when supervised by a trained practitioner.

Notes

_____

_____

_____

_____

_____

_____

_____

_____

_____

_____

_____

_____

_____

_____

_____

_____

_____

_____

_____

_____

Notes

_____

_____

_____

_____

_____

_____

_____

_____

_____

_____

_____

_____

_____

_____

_____

_____

_____

_____

_____

_____

Chapter 10
Breast Cancer: Where are We Now

- Breast cancer

- Signs and symptoms of breast cancer

- Where are we now?
  - Stopping the spread of breast cancer
  - Stool samples can reveal pancreatic cancers earlier
  - Targeting cancer energy supply
  - Making radiotherapy work for more patients
  - Engineering immune cells to hunt down cancer cells

- A mineral capable of destroying breast cancer cells while having no impact on non-cancerous cells

- Topical treatment for breast cancer?

- Pause For Thought

- Take Home Nuggets

- Pages for personal notes

Breast cancer is the most common type of cancer in the UK. Most women are diagnosed after their 50th year, but it can also be found among younger women. This type of cancer not only is present among women, but also occurs in males. It is found a decade later in males, and the presenting signs and symptoms are very similar to those seen in women.

Signs and symptoms of breast cancer include:

a. The presence of a new lump in the breast or under arm (armpit)

b. Thickening or swelling of part of the breast

c. Irritation or dimpling of breast skin (looking like orange peel)

d. Redness or flaky skin in the nipple area or the breast

e. Puckering or pulling in of the nipple or pain in the nipple area

f. Nipple discharge other than breast milk, which may be blood or blood-tinged

g. Any change in the size or the shape of the breast

h. Pain in any area of the breast

These signs and symptoms are not unique to breast cancer, so it is imperative that if you or any of your relatives or friends have these signs and symptoms, please contact your GP/family doctor for a more detailed evaluation.

Where are we now?

As indicated above, there are some gene mutations that increase the risk of breast cancer. We spoke of BRCA1 and BRCA2: these mutations increase the risk of family members with these mutations developing breast/ovarian cancer.

From 2002 Herceptin was made available as a chemotherapeutic agent for treatment of advanced human epidermal growth factor receptor 2 (HER2-positive breast cancer). Interestingly, objective responses were seen in only 15% of patients treated with Herceptin alone, but in an apparent desperate attempt it was rolled out for use nationally. For a mere 15% response, a course of treatment with

Herceptin is estimated at £91,614, based on 3-weekly dose of 3.6 mg/kg for a period of twelve months. It is now emerging that the use of Herceptin for only nine weeks may enjoy better health outcomes, according to new research led by University College London.

The data tells us that with Herceptin plus adjuvant chemotherapy for breast cancer 6.78% more patients are still disease-free who used Herceptin with chemotherapy. An overall estimated median survival is 7.5% higher in the Herceptin with chemotherapy group.

A newer drug available on the NHS used to treat familial breast/ovarian cancer is olaparib. This drug is described as a revolutionary type of targeted anti-cancer medicine called a PolyADP polymerase inhibitors (PARP).

PARP is an enzyme that helps cells repair damaged DNA; by blocking this enzyme in patients, PARP inhibitors prevent the DNA of cancer cells being repaired, preventing them from growing and spreading while leaving healthy cells much less affected. Interestingly, the National Institute for Health and Care Excellence (NICE) opted last year not to recommend olaparib for breast cancer patients with the BRCA mutations because of its high cost, listed at £2,317.50 for one pack of 150 mg tablets, exclusive of VAT, at a dose of 600 mg/day: this allows treatment for only 14 days. This very drug was approved by the Food and Drug Administration for use in the USA in 2014. I note that the reason for NICE refusal was not based on the drug's efficacy but cost. This year we have learned that the drug is now approved by NICE after NHS England struck a deal with AstraZeneca to provide the drug at an undisclosed discount. It is also realised that olaparib has an extensive range of usefulness, being used in the treatment of advanced ovarian cancer, gastric cancer, prostate cancer, pancreatic cancer and of course breast cancer. On average it seems to extend life: the data is encouraging after a 7-year follow-up, with an overall survival of 67% of patients treated with olaparib were alive compared with 46.5% of patients treated with a placebo. I will leave the interpretation of this data to you. My only question is: is treatment patient-driven or money-driven? If money- driven, what becomes of the lives of individuals in the third world?

This, I hear you say, is very expensive for a small benefit, and drives home the recognition that cancer treatment is a very expensive practice with minimal benefits.

Hitherto, most of the emphasis was on the treatment of the condition after it had occurred; the numbers tell of the success or lack thereof from this approach. We have heard of surgery, chemotherapy and radiotherapy as the modalities of treatment since I was in medical school over 30 years ago. Surely our failure in nipping this condition demands that we develop new approaches in this fight. Interestingly the top five developments in 2022 give us a reason to be hopeful. Let's review the top five breakthroughs in the fight against cancer for 2022. Interestingly, there are some new approaches being explored.

1. **Stopping the spread of breast cancer:** Italian scientists have been able to identify a previously unknown way in which breast cancer cells have been able to escape and survive treatment. They found that breast cancer cells hiding in places like the lungs seem to rely on special antioxidants to survive there. This

would give a new approach to wiping out cancer cells which have escaped treatment. The hope is that these findings can be translated into the development of treatment options which can destroy sleeping or dormant cancer cells before they are activated into full-blown metastases.

2. **Stool samples can reveal pancreatic cancers earlier:** Researchers in Spain are now keying in on early detection of pancreatic cancer by sampling stools. They claim that there is a new way to spot if someone is at higher risk of pancreatic cancer and diagnose patients at an earlier stage of this disease and thus increase chances of survival. Specific micro-organisms in stools could signal that there is a problem in a rapid, non-invasive and affordable way. This builds on the growing volume of evidence that the microbiome is linked to the development of cancer.

3. **Targeting cancer energy supply:** Scientists in Germany are now supporting my earlier contention that cutting off the energy supply of cancers could prevent cancers from spreading. Their work, though, seems to be focused on head and neck cancers. If they interfered with required changes in the RNA of mitochondria, the cancer did not spread as much.

4. **Making radiotherapy work for more patients:** Spanish researchers are hopeful that their research could help treat patients who have had cancer spread to their brain. It is felt that in the future a blood test will be able to reveal whether a cancer will respond to radiotherapy or resist it. Additionally, a drug called RAGE inhibitor could make radiotherapy work better for those cancers that would normally resist radiotherapy. The excitement here is palpable

because it raises the probability that this will lead to a new way to personalise the use of radiotherapy and thereby maximise patients' benefits.

5. **Engineering immune cells to hunt down cancer cells:** Researchers in Italy are focused on developing immunotherapy options that could lead to a better and more targeted approach in the fight against cancer. They have already discovered how to engineer a specific type of immune cell that targets and kills cancer cells; the boost is its cancer-killing ability using a drug delivered with nanotechnology. There thus seem to be exciting times ahead in the fight against cancer. The foundation has apparently been laid for an innovative approach of adoptive cell therapy against cancer, which seems to be more efficient than the currently used approaches.

A mineral capable of destroying breast cancer cells while having no impact on non-cancerous cells

Pioneering research in the 1960s and 70s by Dr Eskin repeatedly revealed that iodine is a key element in breast health. Interestingly, iodine kills breast cancer cells without killing normal, non-cancerous cells. It therefore makes it ideal for both treatment and prophylaxis against breast cancer. In one study, Dr Eskin demonstrated that deliberately blocking breast cells from access to iodine resulted in precancerous changes, like that seen when breast cells are exposed to either oestrogen or thyroid hormone. In the absence of iodine, thyroid hormone seems more likely than oestrogen to produce abnormalities in breast cells. Additionally, Dr Eskin was able to show that when breast cells lack iodine, they are more likely to be abnormal, precancerous or cancerous. Iodine-deficient breast tissues are also more susceptible to carcinogen and promote abnormal lesions earlier and in greater numbers. Metabolically, iodine-deficient breasts show changes in RNA/DNA ratios, and oestrogen receptor proteins. Over the past two years research on iodine championed in India and Mexico supports Dr Eskin's original work. These researchers over the past two years have been able to show that iodine supports breast health. It is felt that iodine exerts a suppressive effect on the development and size of both benign and cancerous breast tumours. The researchers in Mexico were able to show in both animal and human studies that molecular iodine supplementation exerts a suppressive effect on the development and size of both benign and malignant neoplasia. Iodine is not only incorporated in thyroid hormones, it is also bound to antiproliferative iodolipids which have anti-cancer activity. In the thyroid gland, these iodolipids are called iodolactones and are believed to play a role in the proliferative control of the mammary gland. They also suggested that breast cancer patients should consider supplementing with iodine in addition to their traditional breast cancer therapy.

The India Research Group demonstrated in 2006 that iodine is toxic to several human breast cancer cell lines.

Topical treatment for breast cancer?

Would it be a considered option of putting the treatment directly unto the problem, the cancer? One suggestion is making a solution of 50% iodine and 50% dimethyl sulfoxide (DMSO) and rub this directly unto the tumour or close to the cancer. The DMSO will ensure penetration deep into the tissue. 70% DMSO solution is readily available, and iodine is available as Lugol's iodine. The mixture can also be rubbed under the armpits to decrease the risk of spread. As indicated above, before embarking on any such treatment, please discuss this with your doctor.

Pause For Thought

- Breast cancer is the most common type of cancer in the UK.
- Most women are diagnosed after their 50th year.
- Breast cancer can also occur in men.
- Signs and symptoms of the disease is similar in both sexes.
- Herceptin has been an expensive disappointment.
- PARP offers the newest hope.
- Top Five breakthrough in cancer treatment of 2022 gives hope.

Take Home Nuggets

- Breast cancer is the most common cancer in the United Kingdom.
- It can affect both men and women.
- The signs and symptoms are similar in both sexes.
- Herceptin is an expensive disappointment.
- There is hope with the new PARP-type preparations.
- We gain further hope from the top five cancer breakthroughs of 2022.
  1. Italian scientist believe that they have found a way to stop the spread of the disease.

2. Spanish investigators believe that they are now able to detect pancreatic cancer at an early stage.

3. German scientists are now able to cut off the energy supply to cancer cells.

4. Spanish researchers are now able to make radiotherapy more effective.

5. Italy researchers using nanotechnology are able to engineer immune cells capable of hunting and killing cancer cells.

6. India research teams are now focussed on treating breast cancer topically.

Notes

_____

_____

_____

_____

_____

_____

_____

_____

_____

_____

_____

_____

_____

_____

_____

_____

_____

_____

_____

_____

_____

Notes

_____

_____

_____

_____

_____

_____

_____

_____

_____

_____

_____

_____

_____

_____

_____

_____

_____

_____

_____

_____

Chapter 11
Pancreatic Cancer

- Pancreatic cancer
- Risk factors for pancreatic cancer
  - Age
  - Smoking
  - Family history of pancreatic cancer
  - Being overweight
  - Pancreatitis
  - Diabetes
- Signs and symptoms of Pancreatic Cancer
- Does stem cell biology provide the answer?
- Pause For Thought
- Take Home Nuggets
- Pages for personal notes

This cancer is both hard to treat and hard to detect, though there seems to be hope on the horizon from the efforts of researchers in Spain, who believe that they are gaining the ability through the assessment of the microbiome in stools to warn of an impending problem with the pancreas and thus facilitate earlier detection of the disease. Until now, patients only experience symptoms after the disease has already spread, which is too late and so today makes it among the deadliest diseases. It has accounted for the lives of the Dirty Dancing movie star, Patrick Swayze, in 2009, and the CEO of Apple, Steve Jobs, in 2011. It is the fifth-biggest cancer killer in the UK; it is the third leading cause of cancer-related deaths in the USA, accounting for 3% of all cancers in the USA; and it has the highest mortality rate of all cancers. It is therefore relatively common. With this data, one cannot sit idly waiting for symptoms to develop, so the approach by our Spanish colleagues in trying to detect the disease earlier is commendable. The best way to beat pancreatic cancer until now is to never get it, which is the best advice in the management of any cancer. In pancreatic cancer, because of the late presentation, by the time you are diagnosed you are given a mere few months to live.

Added to this there is no useful conventional method for treating pancreatic cancer.

Surgery to remove the pancreas is dangerous, so what else is there? As indicated above, by the time the diagnosis is made the cancer has already started to spread, so chemotherapy seems the only option. The available chemotherapeutic options are toxic not only to the cancer cells, but also to normal healthy cells. Unfortunately, this practice has not been shown to improve survival rates, but adds to your symptoms, negatively influencing your quality of life.

Risk factors for pancreatic cancer

There is some evidence suggesting that these factors increase your risk of cancer of the pancreas:

- alcohol

- red and processed meat

- history of cancer

- blood group

- gallstones and gall bladder surgery

Other better-known causes or risk factors for the development of pancreatic cancer include:

Age

As with many other cancers, there seems to be an age association. The risk of developing pancreatic cancer increases with age. In the UK nearly half (47%) of people diagnosed with pancreatic cancer are aged over 75.

Smoking

Smoking cigarettes is associated with pancreatic cancer in about 20% of UK people who have been diagnosed with the disease. One's risk of pancreatic cancer increases the more he/she smokes, and the longer the duration of smoking. Although the evidence on users of e-cigarettes is still being gathered, e-cigarettes are believed to increase the cancer risk twofold.

Around 20 years after stopping smoking, your risk may return to what it would be if you had never smoked.

Being overweight

There is no doubt that being overweight or obese increases the risk of pancreatic cancer. In the UK around one in eight pancreatic cancers (12%) may be linked to being overweight or obese.

Family history of pancreatic cancer

Less than one in ten cases of pancreatic cancers is found to be of a familial type:

- families with two or more first-degree relatives (parent, brother, sister or child) with pancreatic cancer.
- families with three or more relatives with pancreatic cancer on the same side of the family.
- families with a family cancer syndrome and at least one family member with pancreatic cancer. Family cancer syndromes are rare genetic conditions where a faulty gene increases the risk of pancreatic cancer.

Pancreatitis

Inflammation of the pancreas irrespective of the cause is called pancreatitis. This may be associated with spasmodic abdominal pains which may be of variable duration from a few hours to several days, and may worsen with time. This pain may be associated with nausea and vomiting. Over several years, pancreatitis can evolve into symptoms that are linked to difficulty in digesting food. These can mirror some of the symptoms of pancreatic cancer. People with chronic pancreatitis are at increased risk of developing pancreatic cancer.

Diabetes

People with diabetes may have a higher risk of developing pancreatic cancer. But diabetes is common and most people with diabetes won't get pancreatic cancer.

Diabetes can also be a symptom of pancreatic cancer. If you are over 60, have recently been diagnosed with diabetes, and have lost weight without any clear cause, speak to your GP. They should refer you for a scan within two weeks to check for any problems.

This is by no means an exhaustive list and there is some evidence suggesting that these factors increase your risk of cancer of the pancreas.

- alcohol
- red and processed meat
- history of cancer
- blood group: of the four known blood groups A, AB, B and O, it is found that pancreatic cancer is less common among people with blood group O
- gallstones and gall bladder surgery

We have shared repeatedly that apart from never getting cancer, the best way to successfully beat this condition is by diagnosing it early. Above we have indicated that pancreatic cancer presents late, but are there any signs and symptoms that may allow us to discover the disease at an early stage?

Signs and symptoms of pancreatic cancer

Early stages of pancreatic cancer may be asymptomatic. Symptoms will show up only when the disease progresses, and include:

- Digestive problems, including abnormal stools, nausea or vomiting
- Pain in the upper abdomen and back
- Loss of appetite
- Sudden weight loss
- Jaundice (yellowing of the skin and whites of the eyes)
- Very high sugar levels in diabetic patients

Since this disease usually presents in an advanced stage, it is advisable to seek medical attention as early as the commencement of these symptoms suggestive of pancreatic cancer. Hopefully, if the work being pioneered by our Spanish colleagues comes to fruition, this should be a major step in the management and defeat of this ominous disease.

If you or someone you know is exhibiting symptoms of pancreatic cancer, seek medical attention immediately.

Does stem cell biology provide the answer?

The idea that stem cells could play a part in the development of pancreatic cancer and hence its treatment in a large measure was based on the observation of Dr Beard, an embryologist, who made three critical observations about stem cells and their behaviour.

He observed that the stem cells from the placenta had an anatomical makeup that was like cancer cells, but these stem cells exhibited behaviours that were like cancer cells.

These stem cells (a) invade the uterine tissue; (b) build up a vigorous blood supply to support placental growth; (c) proliferate rapidly; and (d) produce human chorionic gonadotropin (hCG).

Based on these observations, Dr Beard came to believe that cancer cells were actually trophoblast stem cells that have broken loose of control mechanisms. Further to this, Dr Beard noted that around day 56 of gestation, the trophoblastic cells lost their malignant characteristics and began to behave like mature foetal cells. Interestingly at about the same time, the foetal pancreas began to show evidence of pancreatic enzymes being produced. It is logical to believe that the transformation in the behaviour of the placental trophoblast and the behaviour of the pancreas may be related and could provide some insight into the appropriate approach to the treatment of this deadly disease.

Emerging from Dr Beard's findings, the Gonzalez Protocol came into being. This protocol is yet to gain widespread acceptance because in clinical studies the results are less than encouraging. I believe, though, that combining the efforts of our Spanish colleagues and the work of Dr Beard and the Gonzalez Protocol there is hope in the future treatment and more successful management of this deadly disease.

Pause For Thought

- Microbiome in stools can help in the early diagnosis of pancreatic cancer.
- In pancreatic cancer, patients only experience symptoms after the disease has spread.
- Cancer of the pancreas is the fifth biggest cancer killer in the UK.
- In the USA, cancer of the pancreas is the third leading cause of cancer related deaths and it has the highest mortality rate of all cancers.
- Treatment options for this disease are limited. Surgery is very dangerous and is not an option for treatment. It would seem that chemotherapy is the only option.
- Several factors are associated with pancreatic cancers and 1in 8 cases of pancreatic cancer is linked to being overweight.
- The Gonzalez Protocol.

Take Home Nuggets

- Pancreatic cancer is usually diagnosed in an advanced state.
- Treatment modality is restricted to chemotherapy as surgical treatment is particularly risky.
- Pancreatic cancer is the fifth biggest cancer killer in the UK, and it is the third leading cause of cancer related deaths in the USA.
- There are several lifestyle factors which are associated with pancreatic cancer such as cigarette smoking and obesity.

Notes

Notes

Chapter 12
Bowel Cancer

- Bowel cancer
- Risk factors for developing bowel cancer
- Pause For Thought
- Take Home Nuggets
- Pages for personal notes

Bowel cancer describes cancer found anywhere in the large bowel which includes the colon and the rectum. It is the fourth most common cancer in the UK, and the second biggest cancer killer. In the USA it is the third most common cancer diagnosed in both men and women. Impressively, the rate of people being diagnosed with colon or rectal cancer each year has dropped overall since the mid-1980s: the reason advanced is more effective screening and changing lifestyle-related risk factors. From 2011 to 2019, incidence rates dropped by about 1% each year. This downward trend is mostly in older adults. In younger people under age 50 years, the rates have been increasing by 1-2% a year since the mid-1990s.

Risk factors for developing bowel cancer

Age again is another risk factor. but other risk factors include:

- Inflammatory bowel disease such as Crohn's disease or ulcerative colitis.

- A personal or family history of colorectal cancer or colorectal polyps.

- A genetic syndrome such as familial adenomatous polyposis (FAP) or hereditary nonpolyposis colorectal cancer (Lynch syndrome).

Lifestyle factors that may contribute to an increased risk of colorectal cancer include:

- Lack of regular physical activity

- A diet low in fruit and vegetables

- A low-fibre and high-fat diet, or a diet high in processed meats

- Overweight and obesity

- Alcohol consumption

- Tobacco use

Main symptoms of bowel cancer include:

a) Changes in your bowel habits: you may experience diarrhoea alternating with constipation which may be unusual for you.

b) There may be a sensation of incomplete emptying with a desire for more frequent emptying of your bowels.

c) Blood may be present in your faeces: this may be bright red or dark red/brown blood.

d) There may be bleeding from the back passage.

e) There may be associated abdominal pains which may be intermittent spasmodic pains simulating trapped wind.

f) There may be bloating.

g) Unintentional weight loss.

h) Easy fatiguability.

These are all symptoms of bowel cancer, but they are not unique to bowel cancer.

Pause For Thought

- Bowel cancer can occur anywhere along the length of the large bowel.
- It is the fourth most common cancer in the United Kingdom and it is the second biggest cancer killer. It is the third most common cancer diagnosed in both men and women.
- The incidence of bowel cancer has dropped among older adults but it is increasing among younger people.
- There are several risk factors for bowel cancer.

Take Home Nuggets

- Bowel cancer occurs in the large bowel including the rectum and anal canal.
- It is the fourth most common cancer in the United Kingdom.
- The incidence has been decreasing among the older generation, but increasing in the younger age groups.

- Risk factors include: Chron's disease, ulcerative colitis, a family history, genetic syndromes, life style factors (diet, obesity, alcohol consumption, tobacco use).

- Signs and symptoms include: change in bowel habits, sensation of incomplete emptying, blood in the faeces, spasmodic abdominal pains, bloating, weight loss and easy fatiguability.

Notes

_____

_____

_____

_____

_____

_____

_____

_____

_____

_____

_____

_____

_____

_____

_____

_____

_____

_____

_____

_____

_____

_____

_____

Notes

Chapter 13
Prostate Cancer

- Prostate Cancer

- CA125 versus PSA

- How Does Ca125 Relate to PSA

- Risk factors for developing prostate cancer

- Symptoms of prostate cancer

- How can this be prevented?

- Improving the Efficiency of Natural Cancer Killers

- ProstaCaid efficiency

- The Combination of ProstaCaid and PectaSol-C

- Pause For Thought

- Take Home Nuggets

- Pages for personal notes

This is a disease of the male subject; females lack a prostate. The prostate is a male sexual organ that produces secretions during sexual arousal. Increasing numbers of men are now being diagnosed with prostate cancer. Additionally, the number of men dying from the disease is also increasing. In the USA, in 2014, it is estimated to have caused more than 29,000 deaths.

To identify the presence of cancer in its very early stages, even before symptoms appear, the United Kingdom has a national screening programme for breast cancer, cervical cancer, and stomach cancer. Sadly, despite the devastation caused by prostate cancer, there is no national screening programme for prostate cancer. The rationale advanced is that we lack a useful, reliable screening tool. The PSA (prostate-specific antigen blood test has been bandied about, but this test has been criticised for not being sufficiently sensitive or specific to be used as a screening tool on which to base a national screening programme.

Recently, there has been reason for hope in that there is a more sensitive tool available. With the advent of magnetic resonance imaging (MRI), specifically the prostate multiparametric (a special MRI for imaging the prostate gland), there is renewed hope that a national screening programme for prostate cancer can be rolled out. It has been found that the pooled sensitivity of MRI in detecting prostate cancer was 89%, with a specificity of 64%. The sensitivity of a test is the ability of that test to correctly identify an individual with the disease as positive. The specificity, on the other hand, describes the ability of a test to correctly identify people without the disease.

It must be emphasised that a biopsy may be the best method of identifying prostate cancer. A biopsy, though, is an invasive procedure with potential complications. This approach though may not be readily accessible to many a doctor, putting it out of the reach of the common man. A less invasive and more readily reliable and available screening tool may be a step in the right direction, and the availability of the MRI as a screening tool may be considered appropriate to raise the prospects of rolling out a national prostate screening programme.

CA125 versus PSA

CA125 (cancer antigen 125) is a blood test widely used to measure the amount of this protein in a woman's blood to determine the likelihood of that patient having ovarian cancer. It is referred to as a tumour marker in medical parlance. Unfortunately, this substance is found in abnormal levels in a number of benign conditions. It has a sensitivity of only 77%, but this may be as low as 50% in stage 1 epithelial ovarian cancers. Nonetheless, it is readily used as a screening test by GPs.

When compared with the PSA, a value of 4.0ng/ml has a sensitivity of 21 % with a specificity of 91%. In the detection of high-grade prostate cancer, the sensitivity was 51 %. One is therefore tempted to argue why CA125 but not PSA; they are both easy blood tests that may provide information to your doctor.

How Does Ca125 Relate to PSA

Ca125 is a marker for ovarian cancer detection. Blood Ca125 levels increase in about 80% of women with ovarian cancer, and it increases in proportion with disease progression. Prostate-specific antigen (PSA) is the most important tumour marker for prostate cancer. PSA, though, is also secreted by normal prostate tissue, and with benign prostatic hyperplasia, false positive results may be had. The same, though, can be said for CA125, which is elevated above 35U/ml, which is considered to be the upper limit of normal. An elevated CA125 (above 35U/ml) can be found in a woman who is menstruating, who has endometriosis, who has fibroids or even inflammation of her peritoneum, inflammation of her liver, inflammation of her lungs, or in heart failure in women.

PSA sensitivity varies between 9% to 33% depending on the patient's age – that is up to 91% of individuals with an elevated PSA do not have prostate cancer. The sensitivity of CA125 for Stage 1 ovarian cancer may be only 50%.

Risk factors for developing prostate cancer

- Advanced age
- Ethnicity, people of colour (African Americans)
- Family history
- Obesity

Symptoms of prostate cancer include:

- A need to pass urine more frequently, often during the night (nocturia).
- A sensation of urinary urgency.
- There may be a sensation of hesitancy: this essentially is difficulty in commencing urination.
- It may be difficult to completely empty the bladder, or the period of emptying the bladder may be prolonged.
- There is poor flow of urine which presents as a weak urinary stream.
- Blood may be present in the urine and/or in semen during ejaculation.

How can this be prevented?

There is a plant-based pigment called quercetin, which may have the answer to fighting and defeating this awful male disease. Quercetin belongs to the group of polyphenols called flavonoids. Polyphenols are the most prevalent group of substances in the plant world. They are responsible for the bright colours, fragrances, and unique taste that we have come to associate with plants. They play an integral role in protecting plants from the harmful effects of ultraviolet radiation from the atmosphere, environmental pollutants, and disease. In studies involving cancer cells, quercetin encourages cancer cells to self-destruct.

Our immune systems react to cancer cell invasions by sending out messages that promote inflammation. Unfortunately, inflammation also promotes tissue damage. In cancer cells, proinflammatory messengers stimulate growth and slow or bypass their natural death process.

Cancer cells need to be in constant communication with each other; various signaling pathways within cancer cells make this possible. Signal transducer and activator of transcription 3 (STAT 3) is a triggered pathway that is one of the main growth-stimulating signals used by cancer cells. Quercetin is believed to be among the agents able to block this STAT 3 pathway most effectively.

Research published in 2015 in the Journal of Oncology Reports revealed several dozen published studies of quercetin and prostate cancer. The conclusion from these studies is that both in vitro (test tubes, petri dishes, outside living organisms) and in vivo (relating to research in living organisms, including human beings), quercetin effectively inhibits prostate cancer in a multiplicity of ways.

Promising results were observed in human clinical trials, and chemopreventative effects such as prevention and slowing of the development of prostate cancer were noted with the use of quercetin in the fight against prostate cancer.

The mechanism by which the STAT 3 pathway is blocked is believed to be related to the impact on messenger IL-6. Quercetin blocks a messenger called interleukin-6 (IL-6). In the presence of cancer, IL-6 activates the STAT 3 pathway; this leads to failure of growth among cancer cells, leading to their eventual death.

Another inflammatory messenger that helps to stimulate prostate cancer growth is called Nuclear Factor Kappa (NF-kappa B). Nuclear factor kappa B is a transcription factor that plays a crucial role in several biological processes, including immune response, inflammation, cell growth, survival, and development. Aberrant NF-kappa B activation contributes to the development of various autoimmune, inflammatory, and malignant tumours. Thus, inhibiting NF-kappa B signaling has potential therapeutic applications in the fight against cancer and inflammatory diseases. A few phenols, as well as quercetin, have been shown to block NF-kappa B, leading to cancer cell death.

Much can be learned from East Asian and Southeast Asian medicine in an attempt to improve western medicine's fight against cancer.

Looking at the incidence of cancer around the world, it is found that the incidence of cancer in the USA is the fifth highest in the world, with an incidence of 352.2/100,000; the sixth-highest incidence is in Belgium at 345.8/100,000; the seventh-highest incidence is found in France with an incidence of 344.1/100000;

the eight highest incidence is found in Denmark with an incidence of 340.4/100000. When these values are compared with those in East Asia and Southeast Asia, with incidence rates in the region of 186/100,000, and Southeast Asia has an incidence of 138.2/100,000; It becomes clear that the incidence of cancer in the Western world is much higher than in East Asia and South East Asia. We may be able to learn from them by studying their lifestyles and understanding why the incidence of cancer in their population is so low. The knowledge gained could help to reduce the incidence of this condition among our people.

A very prominent traditional Vietnamese medicine, so revered in Vietnam that it is reserved for royalty. It was known both as "medicine for the king's palace" and the "royal female herb." This reference is based on the ability of the herb to target both prostate and ovarian health concerns. It, however, appears to be an equal-opportunity herb with benefits beyond the sex-specific diseases. The entry of cucumin in the treatment of ovarian disease is interesting: In 1984, Dr Hong, a medical doctor, treated his daughter, who was preparing to go into surgery for the removal of an ovarian cyst. He allowed her to start drinking tea made from curcumin leaves, and after six weeks, the cysts were all gone.

Improving the Efficiency of Natural Cancer Killers

Prostate cancer is of two types: (a) androgen-dependent cancer and androgen-independent cancer, which has proven to be the more difficult type to treat.

PectaSol-C, developed by the Health Sciences Institute panelist Dr. Isaac Eliaz, is a specialised form of modified citrus pectin (MCP) and has shown great promise against a variety of cancers. In one small study, seven out of ten patients with recurrent prostate cancer significantly slowed their PSA doubling time. PSA can be taken as a measure of how quickly prostate cancer is growing. By reducing the molecular size of the pectin molecule while maintaining its activity against cancers, the product pectaSol-C came into being.

These smaller molecules ensure that more of that pectin can travel through our bloodstream and attack its targets: cancer cells. With this new product, more advanced cancers, including some that had already spread, were successfully treated.

The impressive results seen when patients with prostate cancer are treated with MCP exceed the power of many prescription anti-cancer drugs. There appear to be no dangerous side effects or interactions when MCP is used in treating patients with prostate cancer. Few people have, however, complained of flatulence and loose stool, maybe due to its soluble fibre content. In these situations, one is advised to lower the dose they are on when these side effects are experienced, then gradually work their doses back to therapeutic levels.

Mechanism

We believe from in vitro studies that prostaCaid affects both androgen-dependent and androgen-independent prostate cancer. It is believed that pectaSol-C actually stops the production of new prostate cancer cells and brings on the death of the cancer cells. It seems that in addition to killing off old cancer cells, it is blocking the creation of new ones. It has also been shown that PectaSol-C can work independently, but it is more effective when combined with other prostate cancer-fighting agents.

That group of second cancer-fighting agents is combined in a formula called prostaCaid. ProstaCaid contains an impressive, comprehensive collection of ingredients, thirty-three of the most potent prostate supporters in existence. This complex blend of healing herbs and nutrients provides a wholly integrative approach to conquering prostate cancer. This combination helps not only in promoting but also in maintaining long-term prostate health, which can protect you against the dreaded prostate cancer.

It has been found that the oestrogen/testosterone ratio is crucial to prostate health, and prostaCaid positively balances the oestrogen/testosterone ratio, thus further ensuring prostate health. The ability of this combination of medicines to kill both hormone-sensitive prostate cancer and hormone-resistant prostate cancer (the type that spreads beyond the prostate) is not only remarkable but also unusual. This gives great hope that the specific combination of ingredients can save lives, prevent prostate cancer, and even prolong the lives of those who have prostate cancer.

ProstaCaid efficiency

Both prostaCaid and pectasol-C kill prostate cancer cells through different mechanisms. ProstaCaid actually interrupts the life cycle of prostate cancer cells (a process called G2/M cell cycle arrest).

ProstaCaid cancels or interrupts the cell cycle at the mitosis (cell division) stage. With the prostate cancer cells losing their ability to divide, they die.

ProstaCaid has the same killing effect on androgen-dependent and androgen-independent prostate cancer cells. This is vitally important as, currently, traditional medicine lacks an effective treatment option against hormone-resistant prostate cancer. In trials, it was shown that prostate cancer cell multiplication was stopped, and the cells died after only three days of exposure to ProstaCaid.

ProstaCaid contains about 33 different ingredients; among them is an agent called diinolylmethane (DIM). Dim is a proven cancer-fighting nutrient – specifically as it relates to prostate cancer cells. In mice, it was shown that DIM inhibited prostate tumour growth with no toxic side effects. DIM seemingly inhibits the creation of a particularly dangerous type of oestrogen known as 16α-Hydroxyestrone, instead producing a safer version of the hormone.

Another of the 33 agents in prostaCaid is stinging nettle root. Stinging nettle root is a highly effective cancer substance that can both prevent and treat cancer. Nettle appears to keep benign cells of an enlarged prostate from becoming malignant. Additionally, in vitro studies reveal that stinging nettle can keep prostate cancer cells from multiplying.

The Chinese skull cap is another of the 33 agents in prostaCaid. Chinese Skull Cap, scientifically known as scutellaria baicalensis, has been used traditionally in treating the prostate.

Baicalin is a key compound in Chinese skullcap. This flavonoid inhibits prostate cancer cell growth, whether they are androgen-dependent or not, leading to prostate cancer death. Studies in rodents reveal a 66% reduction in cancer cell mass after just seven weeks of treatment with Chinese skullcap.

Berberine, yet another component of the 33 agents of ProstaCaid, destroys tumours and gets rid of inflammation all at once.

Berberine is an akalloid substance that destroys prostate cancer cells, whether they are androgen-dependent or not. It also keeps cancer cells from multiplying and taking over the organism. It is believed that Berberine works by interrupting the prostate cancer cell life cycle and thus keeps the malignant cells from overtaking the prostate gland. This does not affect healthy prostate cells; it only targets cancer cells.

Pomegranate, yet another component of ProstaCaid, has prostate-saving powers. Numerous studies show how effectively pomegranate fights prostate cancer.

Increased PSA doubling time was recognised among patients consuming eight ounces of pomegranate juice per day. This suggests that this juice has the ability to slow down the aggressiveness of prostate cancer.

In vitro studies using different forms of pomegranate's fermented juice made from the seed prevented prostate cancer cell growth.

Ganoderma lucidum interrupts the cancer supply line, so tumours can't survive. Ganoderma lucidium is also called reishi mushroom. This mushroom has been shown to prevent and induce cell death in prostate cancer cells. It is believed that this mushroom can eventually defeat prostate cancer by cutting off its blood supply. This is achieved by stopping angiogenesis or new blood vessel formation.

In addition, the reishi mushrooms prevent highly aggressive prostate cancer cells from spreading by interrupting special cellular signals, which is integral to getting the cancer under control.

The Combination of ProstaCaid and PectaSol-C

Prostacaid doubles the cancer-killing powers of Pectasol-C; these agents work synergistically in destroying prostate cancer and are much more effective together than individually. It is believed that with both products, the anti-cancer effects of pectaSol-C are doubled.

Using prostaCaid in conjunction with PectaSolC protects the prostate gland. If these two powerful anti-cancer agents cannot be had together and you have to choose one or the other, I recommend ProstaCaid.

Pause For Thought

- Why is the incidence of cancer higher in Western countries than in East and Southeast Asia?

- Could this be because of their diet?

- Is the Japanese herb, the royal female herb, of any benefit?

- Can CA-125 be elevated in the presence of benign conditions?

- Can the CA-125 be raised during menstruation?

- Is the PSA value only raised in the presence of prostate cancer?

- Is PSA value raised in patients with benign prostatic hyperplasia?

- Can prostate cancer be treated with citrus pectin?

- Are there any side effects when using the modified citrus pectin?

- What is the benefit of using both ProstaCaid and pectasolC together in the treatment of prostate cancer?

Take Home Nuggets

- Prostate cancer only occurs in males.

- The incidence of this condition is increasing, as well as deaths from the disease.

- There are several risk factors associated with the development of prostate cancer.

- Prostate cancer is associated with many urinary symptoms.

- Quercetin, a polyphenol, seems to be effective.

- The incidence of cancer in the western countries is higher than in the eastern and southeastern countries.

- It is believed that the difference is based on the difference in diet.

- Modified citrus pectin has been shown to be effective in the treatment of prostate cancer without any significant side effects.

- The major side effects are related to gastrointestinal symptoms such as flatulence and loose motions.

- Pectasol-C works through a variety of pathways.

- Prostacaid is a combination of 33 different ingredients.

- Combining pectasol-C with prostaCaid doubles their effectiveness in the fight against prostate cancer.

Notes

Notes

_____

_____

_____

_____

_____

_____

_____

_____

_____

_____

_____

_____

_____

_____

_____

_____

_____

_____

_____

_____

Chapter 14
Making your Body Cancer-proof

- The carcinogenic toxins

- Infectious causes

- What can we do?

- Pause For Thought

- Take Home Nuggets

- Pages for personal notes

The December edition of the journal *Nature* indicated that researchers from Stony Brook University have confirmed that almost all cancers are caused by factors external to our bodies, which suggests that this can be changed or fixed.

So, by understanding and eliminating some of the commonly known causes of cancer, the disease can be prevented.

The carcinogenic toxins

The toxins are varied and emerge from different sources such as the environment, our behaviour, and infections. Much is known about the relationship of tobacco smoke with lung cancer, but the truth is that every major chemical or heavy metal that we are exposed to is linked to the aetiology of some type of cancer. It therefore stands to reason that the true burden of environmentally induced cancers has been grossly underestimated.

The carcinogenic toxic exposure may be invariably at a low level over an extended period. It seems logical that the prolonged exposure to lower levels of chemicals in the general environment may be contributing to the increasing incidence of cancer.

Infectious causes of cancer

We are familiar with the association between cervical cancer and human papillomavirus. Hepatitis C can cause liver cancer, and the Epstein-Barr virus can cause some forms of lymphoma, a type of cancer which develops in the body's lymphatic system. Helicobacter pylori has been shown to cause stomach cancer. Some gall bladder cancers are associated with salmonella; certain lung cancers may be caused by chlamydial pneumonias, and colon cancer may be caused by three different types of bacteria.

There is also an association between bladder inflammation resulting from some viral infections and prostate cancer, and certain parasites are associated with bladder and bile duct cancers.

What can we do?

Since infectious agents contribute to the development of a range of cancers and, as stated earlier in this section, our immune system plays an integral role in fighting carcinogens., we should take the necessary steps to boost or strengthen our immune systems. Garlic has been known for some time to boost the immune system and it is now known that a high intake of dietary garlic lowers the incidence of both stomach and colon cancers.

We mentioned the plausible role of stem cells in the development of cancer above. There is still much to learn about stem cells. I have actually done some research on stem cells for my dissertation in the completion of my LLM degree. The title of my dissertation was "The legal and ethical basis of stem cells research". We also indicated the similarity in behaviour between stem cells and cancerous growths. We also pointed to a transformation in stem cells behaviour with the advent of thyroid hormones. It is also clear that the ability of the thyroid to produce its hormones by day 45 gestation is without obvious physiological needs, so my question is: could the answer to fighting cancer be tied up with stem cells and understanding how to switch on and off the functionality of these pluripotential cells in the fight against cancer?

As a minimum, we must aim to strengthen our immune system; test for and aggressively treat infections; and rid our environment of heavy metals and known cancer-causing chemicals. The idea of knowingly exposing ourselves to carcinogens, albeit at a low level, will need to be reviewed. So, we need the involvement of our politicians and leaders.

Additionally, the development of vaccines against known oncogenes will be a move in the right direction in the reduction of our body's vulnerability to this condition. We have seen the efficacy of the vaccine against cervical cancer, for example. In a study of almost 1.7 million women with the vaccine against HPV (the virus which causes cervical cancer), it was found that among girls vaccinated before the age of 17, there was nearly a 90% reduction in cervical cancer incidence during the 11-year study period (2006-2017), compared with the incidence among women who had not been vaccinated. Interestingly, as I write, it has recently been indicated in the press that there should be a vaccine available for a variety of cancers by 2035. There is therefore hope on the horizon, because obviously the traditional method of treating cancer through surgery, chemotherapy and radiotherapy has failed and continues to fail us.

Pause For Thought

- Studies show that most cancers are caused by factors external to our bodies.
- To conquer cancer, we need to protect our bodies from the external causes that are known to cause cancer.
- Development of vaccines can help to protect against cancer.
- Evidence for this is seen in the development of the vaccines against HPV the virus which causes cervical cancer.
- This vaccine has led to a 90% reduction in the incidence of cervical cancer.

Take Home Nuggets

- Most cancer are caused by factors outside of our bodies.
- Environmental toxins, infections and behavioural choices can all lead to the development of cancer.
- Heavy metals and chemicals are linked to cancer as a possible cause.

- Exposure to low levels of carcinogens over time can lead to the development of cancer.

- Certain infections can lead to the development of cancer, e.g., HPV can lead to cervical cancer. Hepatitis caused by infections can lead to the development of liver cancer.

- Thus, by boosting our immune system. we may be able to avoid cancer.

- Vaccines may also be useful as the Vaccines against the cause of cervical cancer has been able to reduce the incidence of that disease by 90%.

Notes

_____

_____

_____

_____

_____

_____

_____

_____

_____

_____

_____

_____

_____

_____

_____

_____

_____

_____

_____

Notes

_____

_____

_____

_____

_____

_____

_____

_____

_____

_____

_____

_____

_____

_____

_____

_____

_____

_____

_____

_____

_____

_____

Epilogue

Reclaiming your health is not only possible but necessary if you want to add years to your life and life to your years. Let us explore how this is possible. We look at the 9 most common chronic health issues of today and indicate how these can be overcome. We will explore the disease process, trying to understand their causation, and determine through reliable scientific research how to keep these health challenges at bay. We will also delve into common-sense practices which will play invaluable roles in rendering the disease dormant and in some cases completely reverse the disease process. We encourage the employment of various common-sense measures, as well as provide evidence on how the advised measures work. We are strong proponents of social and preventative medicine and recognise the failure of traditional approaches in the fight against a variety of disease processes.

In this series of 12 books, we will produce easy-to-read manuscripts about each of the nine most common chronic medical conditions, and a book on women's health after the menopause, as well as a book on men's health in which we will question the issue of andropause and address some of the challenges of getting more advanced in age.

With experience and training in organic chemistry, biochemistry and medicine, both as a clinical practitioner and as a trainer for in excess of 30 years, coupled with my years of teaching, I believe that I am uniquely positioned to help you add years to your life and life to your years by attacking and overcoming the vices of modern living which have almost succeeded in overcoming and burdening our very existence through these nine most common chronic ailments. The last three books in this series not only address the issues of getting older, but also suggest methods which you can employ to present the most active versions of yourself even in your twilight years. The final book in this series was empowered by my stem cell research, the legal and ethical issues, during the preparation and fulfilment for the master's degree in law which I was able to complete.

Notes

Notes

www.ingramcontent.com/pod-product-compliance
Lightning Source LLC
Chambersburg PA
CBHW080421030426
42335CB00020B/2535